Summer Desserts for Kids

3rd Edition

29 Recipes to Keep the Kids Cool During the Summer!

by Olivia Rogers

Copyright © 2017 By Olivia Rogers
All rights reserved. No part of this book may be reproduced in any form without permission in writing from the author. No part of this publication may be reproduced or transmitted in any form or by any means, mechanic, electronic, photocopying, recording, by any storage or retrieval system, or transmitted by email without the permission in writing from the author and publisher.
For information regarding permissions write to author at Olivia@TheMenuAtHome.com
Reviewers may quote brief passages in review.

Please note that credit for the images used in this book go to the respective owners. You can view this at:
ArtsCraftsAndMore.com/image-list

Olivia Rogers
TheMenuAtHome.com

Table of Contents

Introduction   5

1. Banana Pudding   6

2. Coconut Cream Pie Bars   8

3. Cool Lemon Bars   10

4. No-Bake Cheesecake   12

5. Coconut-Berry Fro-Yo Pops   14

6. Strawberry Mango Crumble   16

7. Strawberry Margarita Pops   18

8. Banana Bread Ice Cream Sandwich   20

9. Mint Chocolate Chip Ice Cream   22

10. Peanut Butter Pie Pops   24

11. Chocolate Ice Cream   26

12. Chocolate Peanut Butter Banana Icebox Cake   28

13. Lemon-Blackberry Yogurt Pops   30

14. Raspberry Trifle   32

15. Ginger Fruit Salad   34

16. Yogurt with Walnuts & Plum Compote   36

17. Cookie Icebox Cake	38
18. Grilled Peaches with Yogurt	40
19. Key Lime Pops	42
20. Macedonian Fruit Salad	44
21. Macaroon Ice Cream Cake	45
22. Chocolate Muffin Sandwiches	47
23. Ginger Peach Ice Cream Pie	49
24. Raspberry-Orange Sherbet Cake	51
25. Lemon Ices	53
26. Mango Sorbet	54
27. Ice Cream Snow	56
28. Lime Coconut Sorbet	57
29. Creamy Avocado Pops	58
Final Words	60
Disclaimer	61

Introduction

Summer is the perfect season for relaxation but it's also the season for trying every possible way to escape the heat. You can do both of these things with cool, delicious desserts!

This book contains 29 refreshing desserts that will help you cool off while you work on your tan. These recipes are easy-to-make and fun to eat.

Impress your friends with effortless homemade ice creams and sorbets or become the talk of the party by showing up with deliciously cool margarita pops!

Have fun making each of these 29 cool summer desserts!

1. Banana Pudding

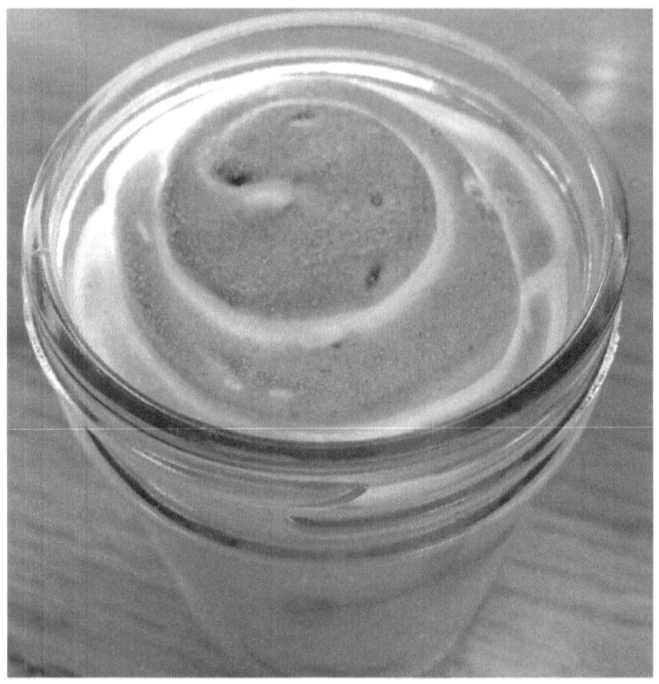

This chilled banana pudding is perfect for a hot summer day.

Ingredients

- About 48 Butter Cookies
- 6-8 Bananas (sliced)
- 2 cups Milk
- 1 (5oz.) box Instant French Vanilla Pudding
- 8 oz. Cream Cheese
- 14 oz. Sweetened Condensed Milk
- 12 oz. Frozen Whipped Topping (thawed)

Method

1. Arrange a layer of butter cookies on the bottom of a baking dish (13"x9"x2"). Arrange a layer of banana slices on top. Blend pudding mix with milk. Beat together cream cheese and condense milk until silky.

2. Whisk in whipped topping. Stir this mixture into the pudding until blended. Pour pudding over bananas. Cover with another layer of butter cookies. Refrigerate 1-2 hours.

2. Coconut Cream Pie Bars

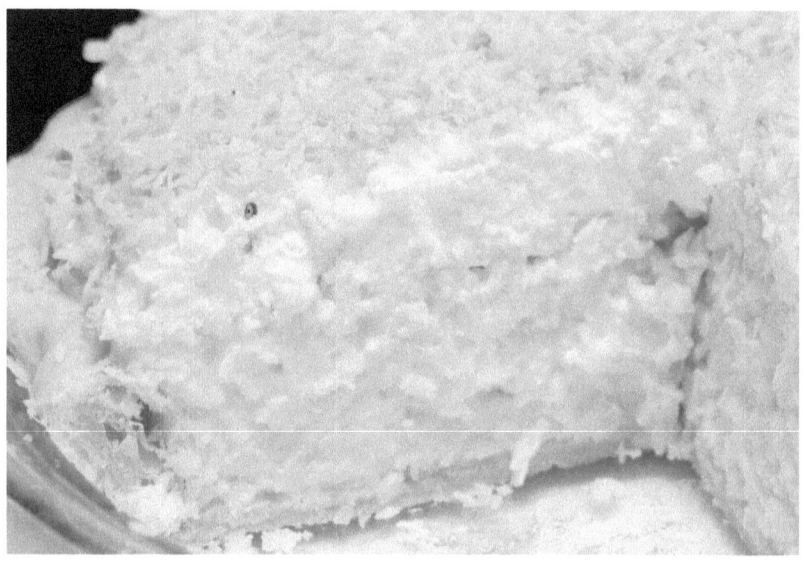

These scrumptious little treats have a refreshing coconut flavor.

Ingredients

- 8 oz. Vanilla Wafers (crushed)
- 24 Vanilla Wafers
- 6 Tbsps. Butter (melted)
- 8 oz. Cream Cheese
- ¼ cup Sugar
- 3 cups Whipped Cream (divided)
- 1 (5oz.) box Vanilla Pudding (prepared)
- 1 ½ cups Coconut Flakes (toasted, divided)

Method

1. Mix together crushed wafers with butter until combined. Spread across the bottom of a baking dish (9"x13") in an even layer. Let set in the fridge. Beat together cream cheese and sugar until smooth. Gradually whisk in 1 cup whipped cream. Spread over chilled crust. Arrange a row of wafers around the edge of the dish (with wafers standing upright). Return to fridge.

2. Whisk together pudding and 1 cup whipped cream. Carefully fold in ¾ cup coconut flakes until just combined. Spread this evenly over the cream cheese layer. Spread remaining 1 cup whipped cream evenly over pudding layer. Sprinkle remaining coconut flakes on top. Let chill 6 hours. Cut into bars to serve.

3. Cool Lemon Bars

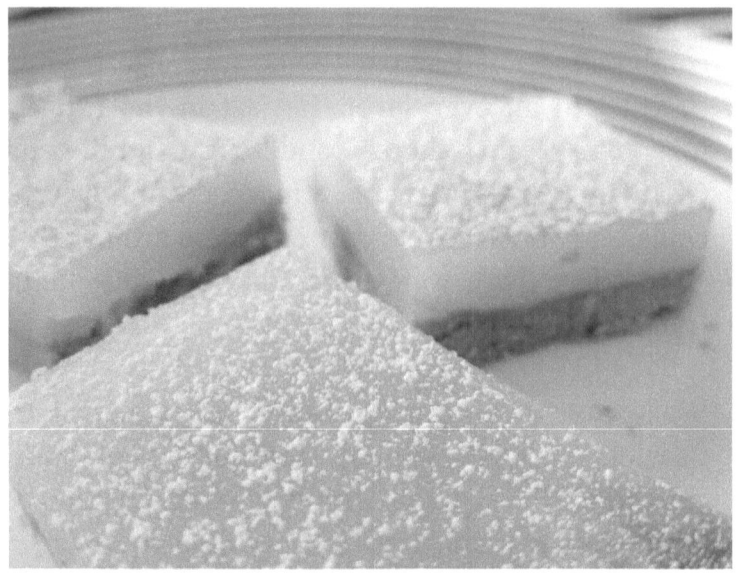

These citrusy sweets get a wonderfully crunchy texture from chopped hazelnuts in the crust.

Ingredients

- 1 cup Butter (softened)
- 2 cups flour
- ¾ cup Powdered Sugar
- ½ tsp Vanilla Extract
- ¼ cup Chopped Hazelnuts
- 1 Tbsp. Fresh Grated Ginger
- ¼ tsp Salt
- 1 Egg Yolk
- 8 oz. Cream Cheese
- 8 oz. Mascarpone Cheese

- 28 oz. Sweetened Condensed Milk
- 4 Large Eggs
- 1 Tbsp. Lemon Zest
- 1 cup Fresh Lemon Juice
- 6 Tbsps. Boiling Water
- 1 Tbsp. Unflavored Gelatin

Method

1. Preheat oven to 350°F. Line a baking dish (9"x13") with aluminum foil. Allow 2" of aluminum to hang over each short side. Beat together butter, sugar, and vanilla until creamy. Gently beat in flour, ginger, salt and egg yolk. Stir in hazelnuts until combined. Spread across bottom of pan in an even layer. Bake 10-15 minutes. Let cool.

2. Beat together cream cheese and mascarpone until creamy. Add condensed milk until blended. Add one egg at a time, beating each well. Add lemon juice and zest. Beat until thickened.

3. In a small bowl, whisk together gelatin and boiling water until dissolved. Let cool 5 minutes. Beat gelatin into lemon mixture. Pour mixture into dish. Refrigerate 8 hours. Cut into bars.

4. No-Bake Cheesecake

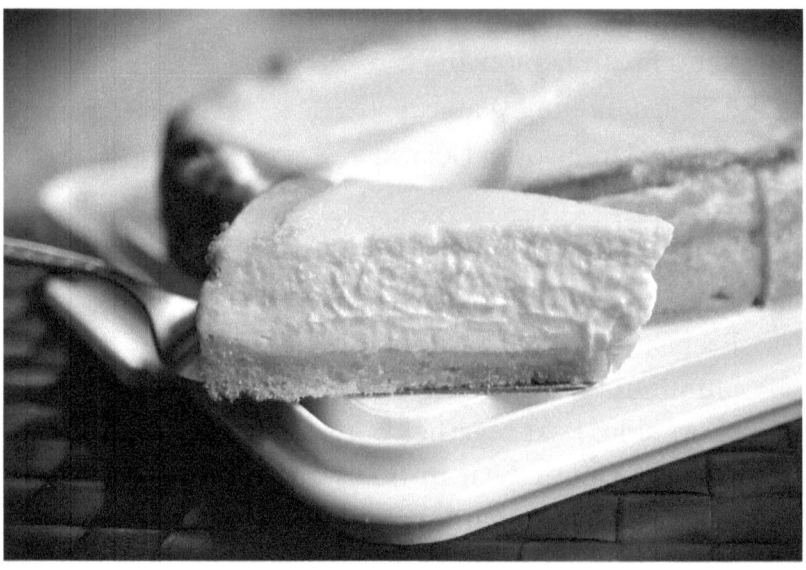

This effortless cheesecake is bursting with fresh blueberry flavor.

Ingredients

- 5 oz. Vanilla Wafers (crushed)
- 4 Tbsps. Butter (melted)
- 8 oz. Cream Cheese
- ¾ cup Sugar
- 1 tsp Vanilla Extract
- Zest from 1 Lemon
- 2 ½ cups Blueberries
- Whipped Cream and more Blueberries to serve

Method

1. Mix together crushed wafers and butter until combined. Divide mixture between 4.5" pie dishes. Press into an even layer on bottom and along sides (about halfway up the sides). Freeze 30 minutes.

2. In a processor, pulse together cream cheese, lemon zest, sugar, and vanilla until smooth. Add blueberries. Pulse until blended. Divide filling evenly between each dish. Cover and chill overnight. Serve with a dollop of whip cream and blueberries on top.

5. Coconut-Berry Fro-Yo Pops

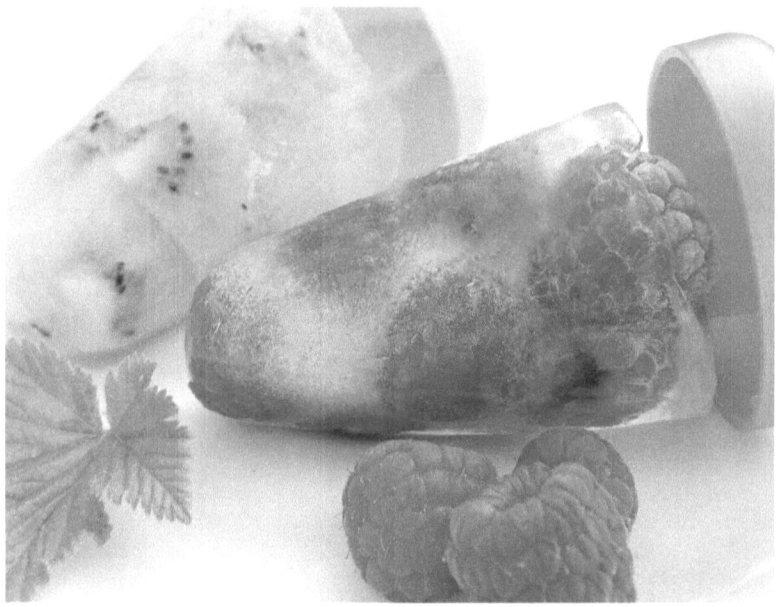

Frozen yogurt is already a great summer dessert, but these Popsicle versions make it an even more fun and convenient treat.

Ingredients

- 2 cups Mixed Berries
- ¼ cup Sugar
- Juice from 1 Lemon
- 1 cup Plain Greek Yogurt
- ½ cup Powdered Sugar
- 1 Tbsp. Coconut Extract
- ½ cup Unsweetened Coconut Flakes

Method

1. In a processor, pulse together first 3 ingredients until smooth. In a bowl, whisk together next 3 ingredients until smooth.

2. Pour alternating layers of berry mixture and yogurt mixture in Popsicle molds. Insert sticks. Freeze 8 hours. Remove from mold and dip into coconut flakes before serving.

6. Strawberry Mango Crumble

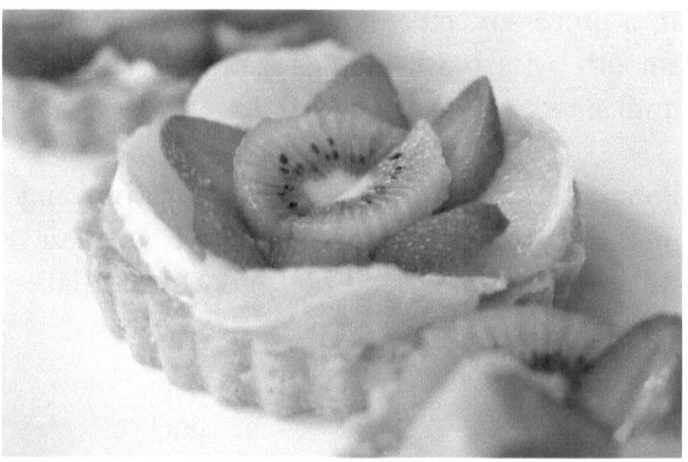

This simple dessert has all the flavors of summer.

Ingredients

- 3 Mangos (peeled, sliced)
- 2 cups Strawberries (quartered)
- 1 Tbsp. Sugar
- 2 Tbsps. Fresh Lemon Juice
- 1 ¼ tsp Cinnamon (divided)
- ¼ tsp Nutmeg
- 1 tsp Grated Ginger
- 3 Tbsps. Flour
- Salt
- 1 ½ cups Flour
- 1 ½ cups Rolled Oats
- 1 cup Brown Sugar
- 10 Tbsps. Butter (softened)

Method

1. Preheat oven to 375°F. Gently mix together strawberries, mangos, 1 teaspoon cinnamon, nutmeg, ginger, 3 tablespoons flour, lemon juice, and a dash of salt. Pour into a deep pie dish (9").

2. In a bowl, stir together oats, brown sugar, flour, a pinch of salt and remaining cinnamon until mixed. Gently massage butter in with a fork until clumpy. Spoon crumbly mixture over fruit filling. Bake 1 hour. Serve with ice cream.

7. Strawberry Margarita Pops

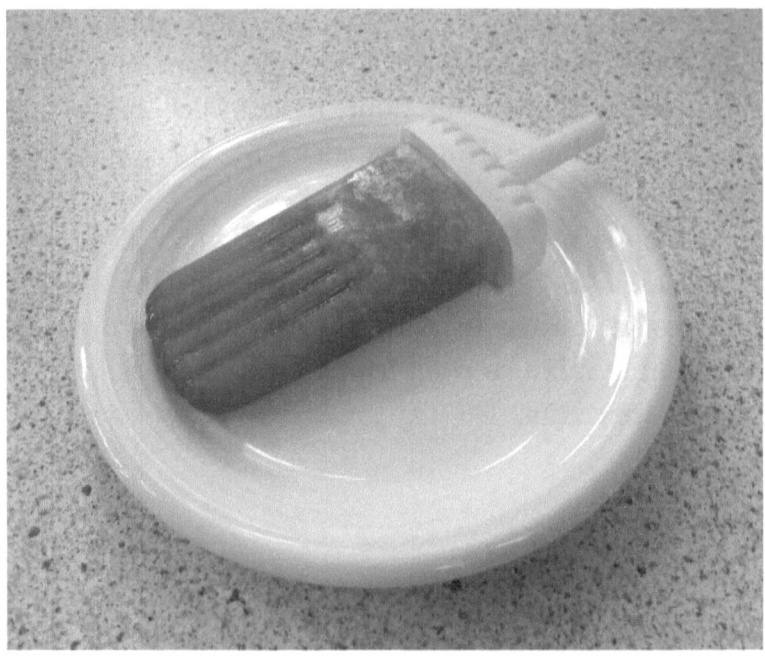

Liven up your backyard barbecue with these fun margarita pops.

Ingredients

- 1 cup Fresh Lime Juice
- ½ cup Water
- ½ cup Triple Sec
- ¼ cup Tequila
- ½ cup Sugar
- 1 pine Strawberries (quartered)

Method

1. Blend together water, triple sec, lime juice, tequila, and sugar until dissolved. Set aside 8 pieces of strawberry. Add rest to blender. Pulse until smooth.

2. Stick a strawberry piece on the end of each Popsicle stick. Pour margarita mix into Popsicle molds. Insert sticks (strawberry side first). Freeze 4 hours.

8. Banana Bread Ice Cream Sandwich

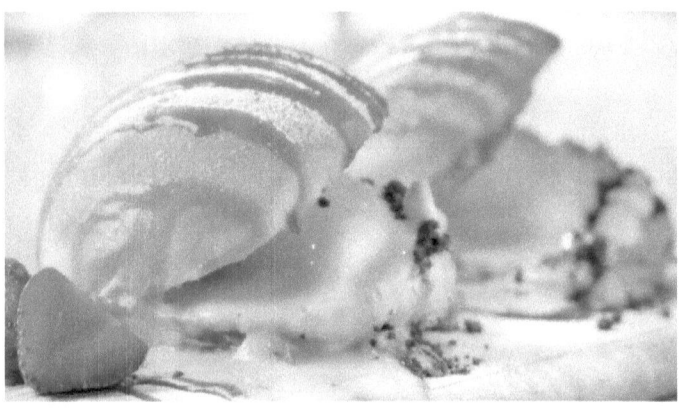

This recipe puts a twist on two classic desserts: banana bread and the ice cream sandwich.

Ingredients

- 3 ripe Bananas
- 1 ½ cups Flour
- 1 tsp Baking Soda
- ¾ tsp Salt
- 2 Eggs
- ½ cup Sugar
- ½ cup Butter (melted)
- 2 Tbsps. Olive Oil
- ½ cup Buttermilk
- 1 ½ tsp Vanilla Extract
- Ice Cream (your choice, or use one of the ice cream recipes in this book)

Method

1. Preheat oven to 350°F. In a bowl, mash bananas until smooth. Whisk in buttermilk and vanilla extract. In a separate bowl, whisk eggs, sugar, butter, and oil until frothy. Stir banana mixture into egg mixture.

2. In another bowl, mix together flour, salt, and baking soda until blended. Gradually add flour mixture to banana mixture until combined. Pour into a greased loaf pan. Bake 1 hour. Let cool.

3. Prepare a grill for medium-high heat. Cut banana bread into 16 slices. Grill slices 2-3 minutes per side. Let cool. Spread about 1 cup of ice cream evenly on each sandwich to make 8 sandwiches. Chill sandwiches 1 hour.

9. Mint Chocolate Chip Ice Cream

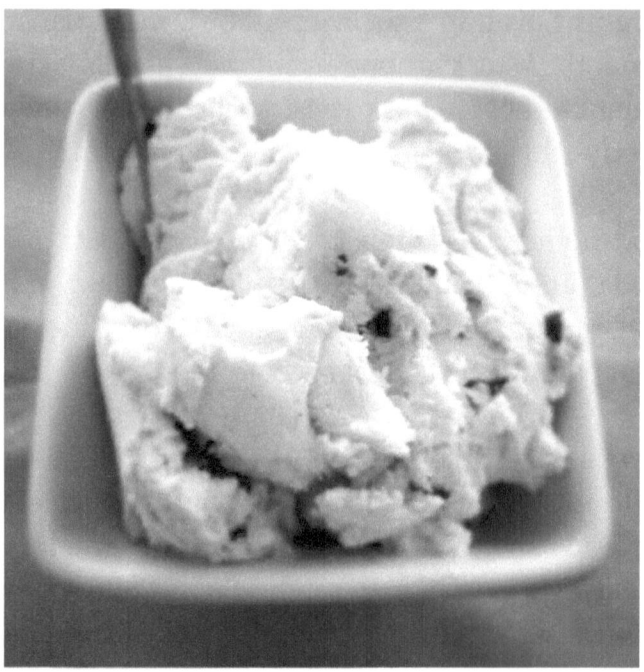

Make this classic summer treat from scratch in your own kitchen!

Ingredients

- 3 cups Half & Half
- 1 cup Heavy Cream
- 8 large Egg Yolks
- 9 oz. Sugar
- 1 tsp Peppermint Oil
- 3 oz. Dark Chocolate (chopped)

Method

1. In a medium over medium heat, stir together cream and half & half until simmering. Remove from heat. In a bowl, whisk egg yolks until they lighten. Slowly whisk in sugar. Add 1/3 of cream mixture in spoonful until well blended. Pour in the rest of the cream in one batch.

2. Return mixture to the pot and place on low heat. Stir often until mixture thickens. Pour into a bowl and let rest 30 minutes. Stir in peppermint oil. Chill in fridge 4-8 hours (until mixture is 40°F. Pour mixture into an ice cream maker with dark chocolate. Prepare according to directions.

10. Peanut Butter Pie Pops

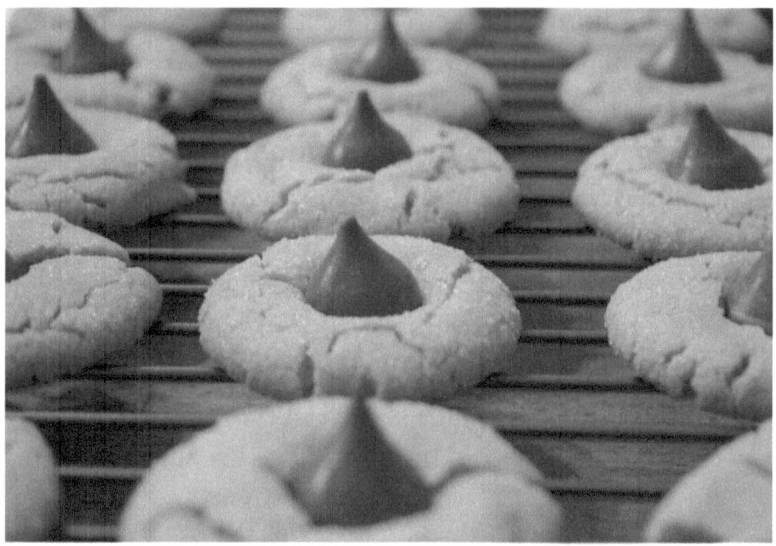

These peanut butter pie pops are both satisfying and refreshing.

Ingredients

- ½ cup Graham Cracker Crumbs
- ¼ cup Pretzels (crushed)
- ¼ cup Sugar
- 1 Tbsp. Cocoa Powder
- 3 Tbsps. Melted Butter
- 12 oz. Cream Cheese
- 8 oz. Peanut Butter
- 4 oz. Powdered Sugar
- ½ tsp Salt
- 1 tsp Vanilla Extract
- ¼ cup Roasted Peanuts (chopped)

- 1 ½ cups Heavy Cream
- ½ cup Toffee Pieces
- 6 oz. Dark Chocolate (chopped)

Method

1. In a bowl, mix together first 4 ingredients. Mix in butter until combined. Beat cream cheese until smooth. Beat in next 4 ingredients until mixture is light and fluffy. Stir in peanuts until evenly distributed.

2. In another bowl, whip heavy cream into firm peaks. Fold cream into peanut butter mixture in ½ cup batches. In the Popsicle mold, add alternating layers of peanut butter mixture, toffee pieces, chocolate, and graham cracker mixture until filled. Insert sticks. Freeze overnight.

11. Chocolate Ice Cream

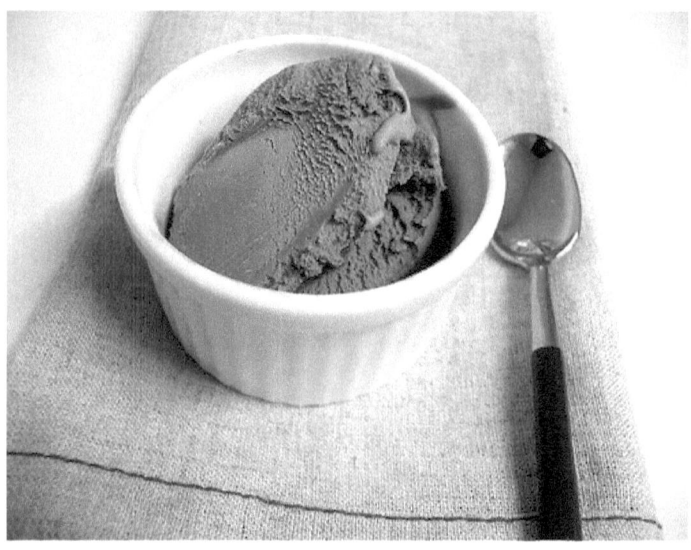

Make your own sinfully delicious chocolate ice cream with this recipe.

Ingredients

- ½ cup Unsweetened Cocoa Powder
- 3 cups Half & Half
- 1 cup Heavy Cream
- 8 large Egg Yolks
- 9 oz. Sugar
- 2 tsp Vanilla Extract

Method

1. In a medium pot over medium heat, whisk together 1 cup half & half with cocoa powder until combined. Add

cream and remaining half & half. Stir just until simmering. Remove from heat.

2. In a bowl, whisk yolks until lightened. Slowly whisk in sugar. Whisk cream into the egg mixture in 1/3 cup batches. Pour back into pot. Place over low heat. Stir until mixture thickens. Pour into a bowl. Let rest 30 minutes.

3. Stir in vanilla extract. Cover and chill 4-8 hours (until mixture is 40°F). Pour into an ice cream mixer and prepare according to directions.

12. Chocolate Peanut Butter Banana Icebox Cake

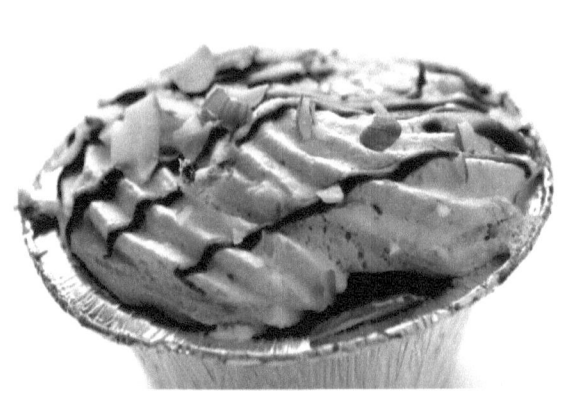

This no-bake cake combines the rich flavors of peanut butter, chocolate, and banana.

Ingredients

- ½ cup Peanut Butter
- 2 ½ cups Heavy Cream (chilled, divided)
- ½ cup Powdered Sugar
- 1 ½ tsp Vanilla Extract
- 5 ripe Bananas (sliced)
- 2 (9oz.) packages Chocolate Wafer Cookies

Method

1. In a large bowl, whisk together peanut butter and ½ cup cream until fluffy. Set aside.

2. In a separate bowl, whip remaining cream with sugar and vanilla extract to firm peaks. Fold about ½ cup whipped cream into peanut butter mixture. Add peanut butter mixture into whipped cream in 3 batches until well combined. Set aside.

3. Arrange a layer of wafers in a 9" pie dish. Spread a layer of peanut butter mixture on top. Add a layer of banana slices. Repeat layering until ingredients are used. Cover and chill 4 hours.

13. Lemon-Blackberry Yogurt Pops

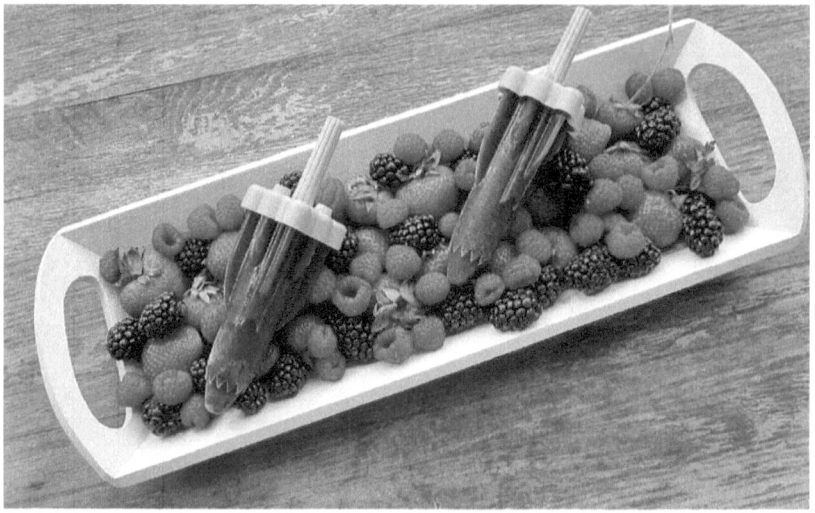

These cool popsicles are a perfect balance of tangy and sweet.

Ingredients

- 1 Lemon
- ½ cup Water
- ½ cup Sugar
- 1 ½ cups Plain Greek Yogurt
- 2 cups Blackberries (halved)

Method

1. Peel off yellow layer of lemon. Set lemon aside for another use. In a small pot over medium-high heat, stir together water and sugar until dissolved. Gently stir in lemon peels. Simmer 5 minutes. Let cool.

2. Strain syrup into a bowl. Chill. Stir yogurt into syrup until well combined. Stir in blackberries. Fill Popsicle molds with yogurt mixture. Insert sticks. Freeze 3-4 hours.

14. Raspberry Trifle

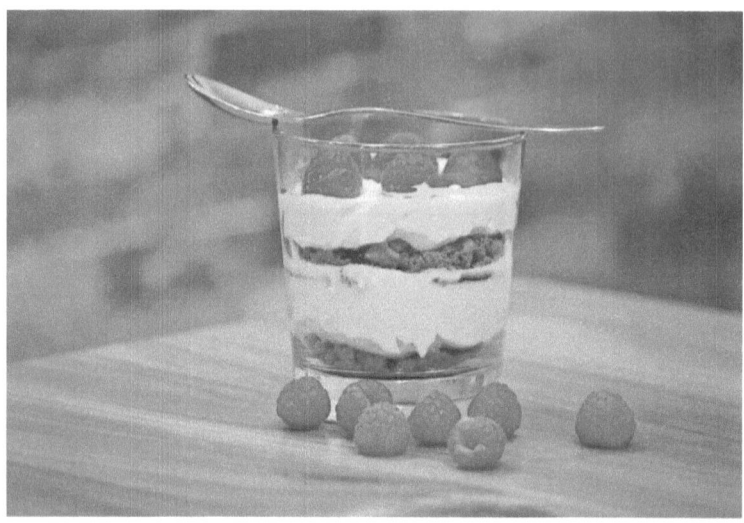

This simple custard dish is bursting with cool raspberry flavor.

Ingredients

- 9 Egg Yolks
- 4 cups Whole Milk
- ½ cup Sugar
- ½ Vanilla Bean (seeded)
- ¼ cup Water
- 1 cup Raspberry Jam
- 1 cup Heavy Cream
- 1 cup Dry Sherry
- 2 loaves Pound Cake (sliced)
- 3 cups Frozen Raspberries (defrosted)
- 2 cups Fresh Raspberries

Method

1. In a bowl, whisk together milk, yolks, ¼ cup sugar, and vanilla seeds. Pour into a double boiler and set over medium heat, whisking constantly for 30 minutes without letting it boil. Refrigerate 2 hours.

2. Bring water to a boil in a small pot. Remove from heat. Stir in jam. Dip one side of each pound cake slice into the sherry. Arrange a layer of pound cake on the bottom of a large clear bowl.

3. Pour a thin layer of custard over the slices (just enough to cover). Spoon in a few teaspoons of jam. Sprinkle in some defrosted raspberries. Repeat layering until ingredients are used. Poke a knife through the top in a few places. Top with fresh raspberries and whipped cream (if desired). Chill 1 hour.

15. Ginger Fruit Salad

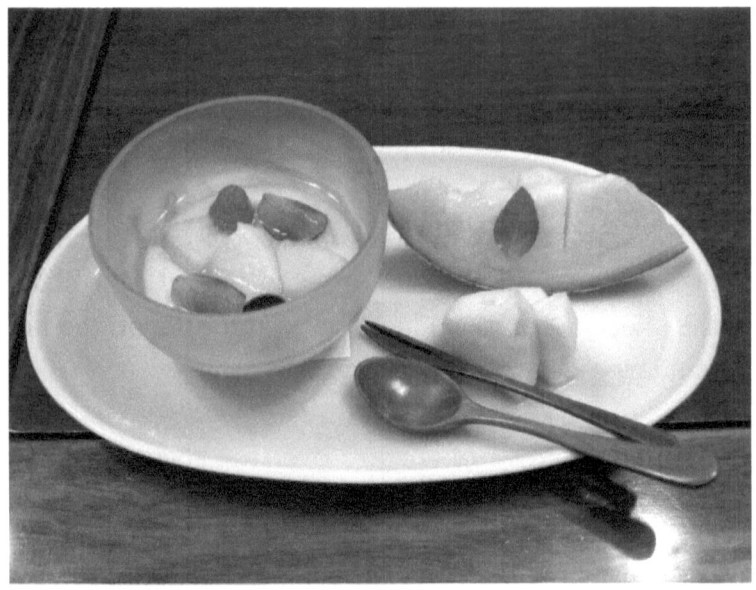

This jazzed up fruit salad is brimming with tropical flavor.

Ingredients

- ¼ cup Sugar
- 1 (3") piece Ginger (peeled, chopped)
- Zest from 1 Lime
- 1-pint Strawberries (quartered)
- 2 Kiwis (peeled, quartered)
- 1 Mango (cut into chunks)
- 1 Pineapple (cut into chunks)
- 1 Papaya (cut into chunks)
- 1 handful Fresh Mint (chopped)

Method

1. In a small pot, boil water, lime zest, ginger, and sugar until dissolved. Remove from heat. Refrigerate until chilled.

2. Strain syrup into a large bowl. Add fruits. Toss to coat. Chill 1 hour. Garnish with fresh mint before serving.

16. Yogurt with Walnuts & Plum Compote

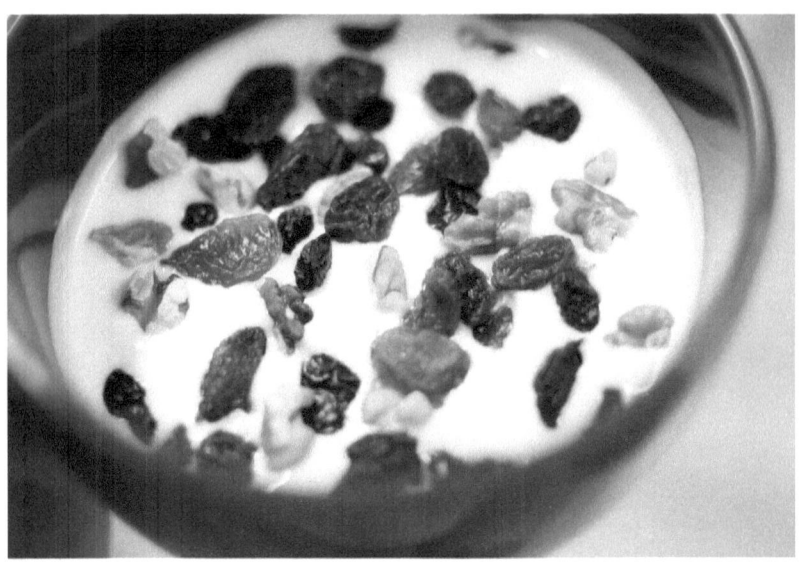

Yogurt gets a makeover with this irresistible plum and walnut topping.

Ingredients

- 5 Ripe Plums (pitted, quartered)
- 3 Tbsps. Maple Syrup
- 2 Tbsps. Water
- Juice from ½ Lemon
- 1 Cinnamon Stick
- 1 ¼ cups Toasted Walnuts
- 6 cups Vanilla Greek Yogurt

Method

1. In a pot over medium-low heat, cook plums, lemon juice, maple syrup, water, and cinnamon stick. When simmering, stir and reduce heat to low. Let cook 15 minutes. Remove from heat.

2. Stir in 1 cup walnuts. Divide yogurt into bowls. Spoon plum compote over the top. Sprinkle with remaining walnuts.

17. Cookie Icebox Cake

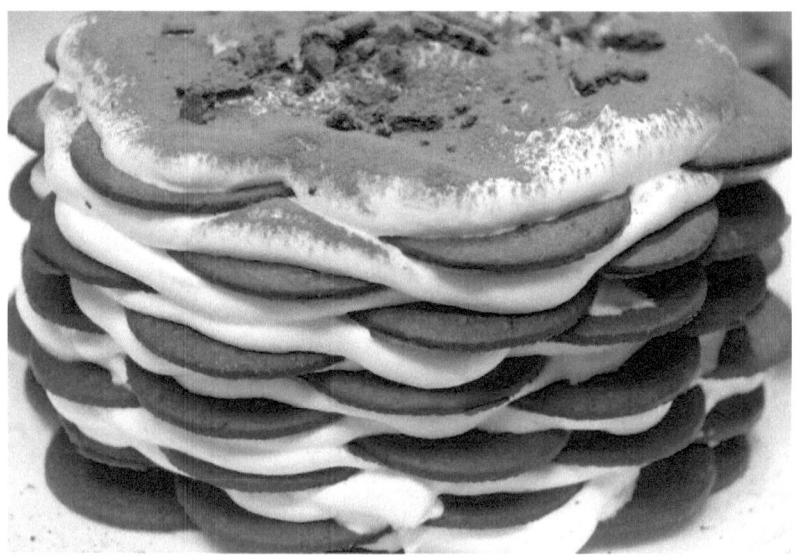

This simple no-bake cake is perfect to whip up for a potluck or barbecue.

Ingredients

- 40 Chocolate Wafer Cookies
- ¾ cup Sugar
- ¼ cup Water
- 3 cups Whip Cream

Method

1. Pour sugar into a medium pot so that it forms a pile in the center. Slowly add water without letting sugar hit the sides of the pan. Cook over high heat. When sugar

starts to color, gently stir. Let it become dark. It will smoke a bit.

2. Once darkened, reduce heat to medium-low and add 1 ½ cups cream. Gently whisk until caramel dissolved. Stir in remaining cream. Strain into a bowl. Cover and chill. Whisk 2/3 of the chilled caramel cream to soft peaks.

3. Line a loaf pan (8"x4") with plastic wrap. Add a layer of cream to the bottom. Add a layer of cookies. Repeat layering until ingredients are used. Chill 3 hours. Invert cake onto a platter. Whip remaining cream into firm peaks. Spread over the cake.

18. Grilled Peaches with Yogurt

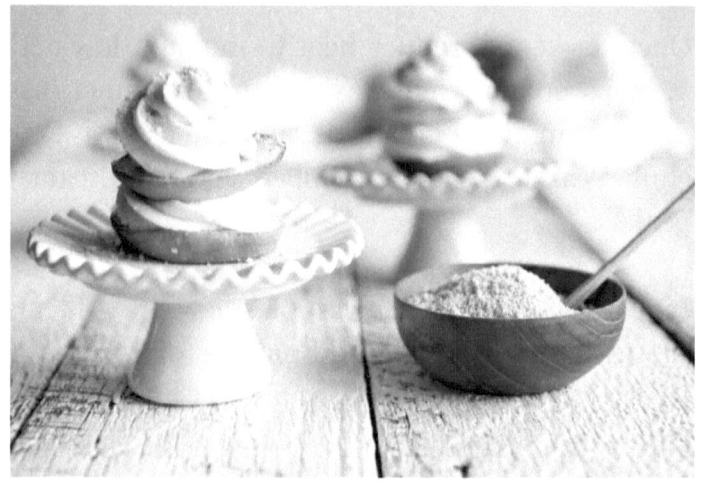

This dessert is healthy and elegantly simple to make.

Ingredients

- 12 Peaches (halved, pitted)
- 2 Tbsps. Olive Oil
- Salt
- 2 cups Plain Greek Yogurt
- ¼ cup Honey
- 1/" cup Fresh Mint (chopped)

Method

1. Prepare grill for high heat. Brush oil on peach flesh. Sprinkle lightly with salt. Place peaches (flesh-side down) on grill. Cook 1-2 minutes.

2. Transfer to plates and serve with a large dollop yogurt. Drizzle over with honey and sprinkle on fresh mint.

19. Key Lime Pops

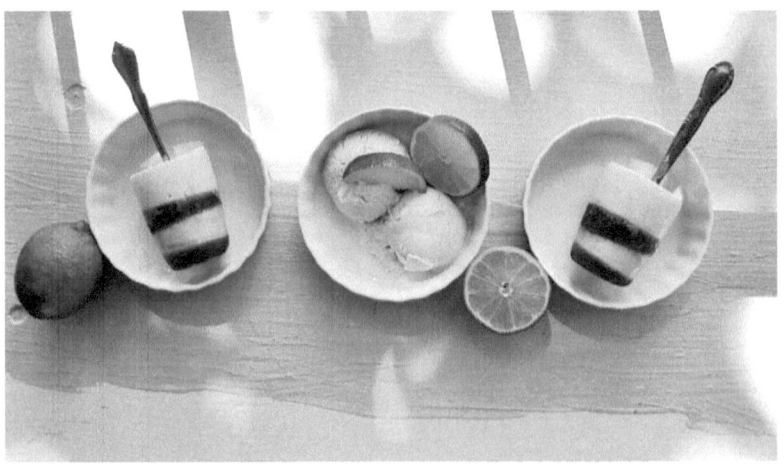

This recipe gives you a cool new way to enjoy the refreshing flavor of key lime pie.

Ingredients

- 1 (14oz.) can Sweetened Condensed Milk
- 1 cup Half & Half
- ¾ cup Fresh Lime Juice
- 2 tsp Lime Zest
- Salt
- 3 cups Graham Crackers Crumbs

Method

1. In a bowl, whisk together first 5 ingredients until well combined. Divide mixture into Popsicle molds. Freeze 1 ½ hours. Insert sticks. Freeze 4 hours.

2. Spread graham cracker crumbs on a plate. Press popsicles into crumbs until coated on all sides.

20. Macedonian Fruit Salad

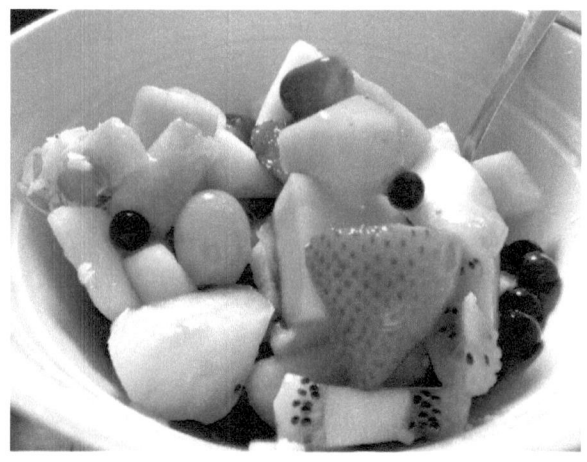

Enjoy this healthy Mediterranean-inspired version of the classic fruit salad.

Ingredients

- 1 lb. Strawberries (quartered)
- ½ lb. Blueberries
- ½ lb. Blackberries
- ½ lb. Raspberries
- Juice from 3 Oranges
- Juice from 1 Lemon
- 1 Handful Fresh Mint (chopped)

Method

1. In a large bowl, mix berries together. Add orange and lemon juice. Stir to coat. Cover and chill 2 hours.

21. Macaroon Ice Cream Cake

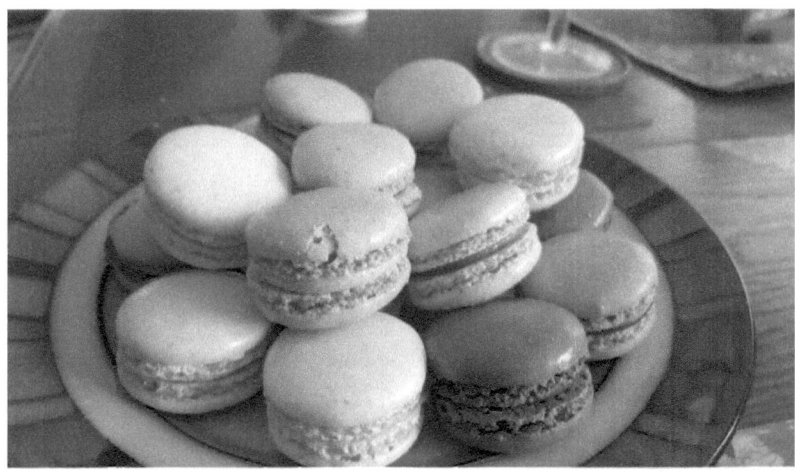

This coconut-chocolate treat is a sweet way to cool off this summer.

Ingredients

- 2 pints Chocolate Ice Cream (try using recipe in this book)
- 2 pints Vanilla Almond Ice Cream
- 1 package Soft Coconut Macaroons
- ½ cup Chocolate Shell Ice Cream Topping
- 1 cup Sliced Almonds

Method

1. Lightly grease a baking dish (8"x3") with butter. Crumble half of the macaroons. Spread across the bottom of the dish (and about 1" up the sides). Spread a

layer of chocolate ice cream evenly on top of macaroon crust.

2. Crumble remaining macaroons. Spread evenly over chocolate ice cream. Freeze 45 minutes. Spread a layer of vanilla almond ice cream on top. Let freeze 4 hours.

3. Pour chocolate topping on top of cake. Tilt dish to spread coating across the top. Let harden. Wrap a damp, warm towel around pan to loosen sides. Remove cake. Press sliced almonds onto the sides.

22. Chocolate Muffin Sandwiches

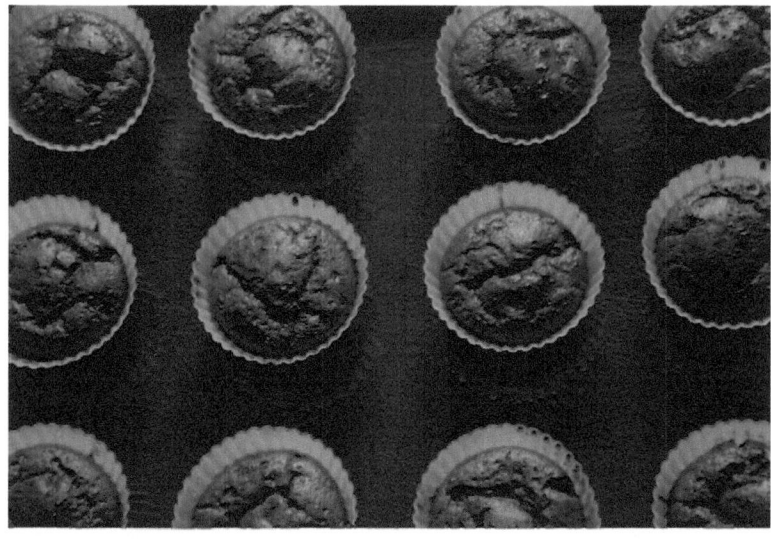

Chocolate muffins and ice cream combine for a simple and delicious dessert.

Ingredients

- 1 cup (+ 6 Tbsps.) Vanilla Ice Cream
- 4 Chocolate Chip Muffins
- 4 large Strawberries (sliced)

Method

1. Use a small ice cream scoop to scoop out 4 ice cream balls. Set on plate and store in freezer. Cut muffins in half horizontally. Press a small indentation in the cut side of the bottom piece with a spoon.

2. Melt 1 cup ice cream in a small pot over low heat, stirring often. Place one ball ice cream in each indent made in the muffin bottoms. Place the muffin top on and spoon over with melted ice cream. Sprinkle with strawberries.

23. Ginger Peach Ice Cream Pie

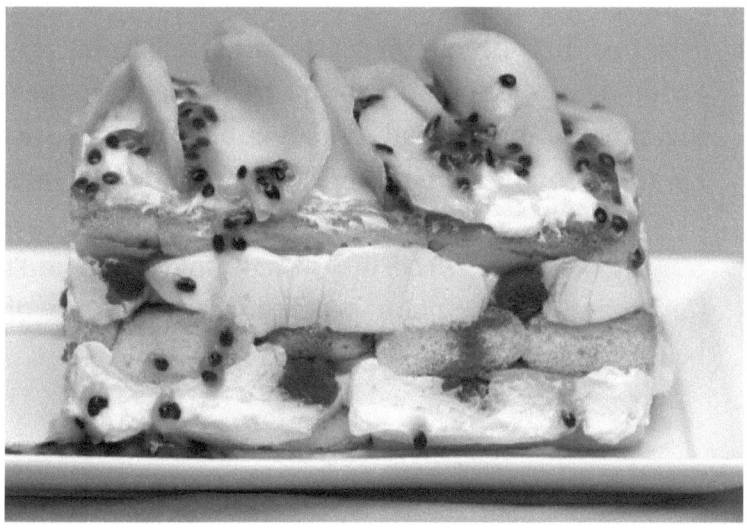

This pie recipe is light and refreshing—perfect for a hot summer day.

Ingredients

- 12 Cinnamon Graham Crackers (crumbled)
- 5 Tbsps. Butter
- 1/3 cup Chopped Crystallized Ginger
- 1 ½ cups Peach Preserves
- 8 cups Peach Ice Cream
- 1 Peach (thinly sliced)

Method

1. Lightly grease a 9" pie dish. Mix together graham cracker crumbs, butter, and 2 tablespoons ginger until

combined. Spread crumb mixture in an even layer across bottom and sides of dish. Freeze 30 minutes.

2. Stir together peach preserves and remaining ginger. Scoop 4 cups ice cream into pie dish. Place scoops close together. Do not spread. Pour 1 cup peach mixture over the top. Scoop in remaining ice cream. Freeze 3 hours.

3. Stir fresh peach slices into remaining peach mixture. Cover and chill. Spoon peach mixture on top of pie before serving.

24. Raspberry-Orange Sherbet Cake

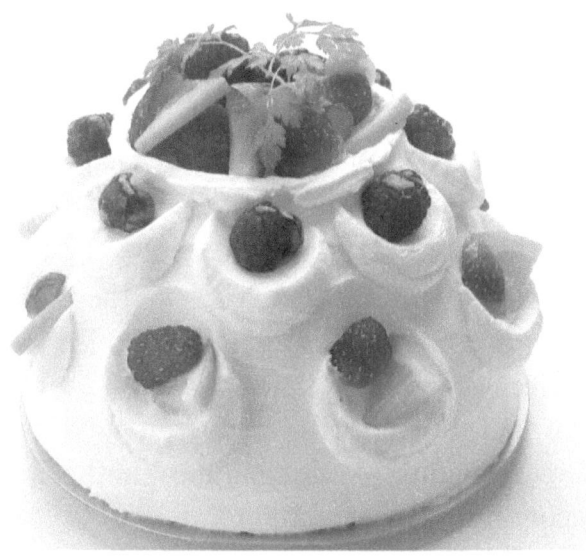

Raspberry and orange ice cream give this cake a sweet tangy touch.

Ingredients

- 2 packages Coconut Macaroons
- 3 cups Raspberry Sherbet
- 2 pints Vanilla Ice Cream
- 3 cups Orange Sherbet
- 1 Orange (peeled, sliced)
- 2 cups Raspberries
- ½ cup Water
- ½ cup Sugar

Method

1. In a pot over medium-high heat, stir together water and sugar until dissolved. Stir in orange slices and raspberries. Bring to a boil. Let cook 10 minutes. Remove from heat. Set aside. Line a baking dish (13"x9") with foil. Allow 2" foil to hang over each short side. Lightly grease with butter.

2. Arrange a layer of macaroons on the bottom of the dish. Drop in spoonsful of sherbets and ice cream. Alternate flavors and pack down as you go until bottom is covered. Spread a layer of fruit mixture over the top. Freeze 2 hours. Add remaining sherbet and ice cream in spoonful. Freeze 30 minutes. Add remaining fruit mixture and another layer of macaroons. Freeze 6 hours.

25. Lemon Ices

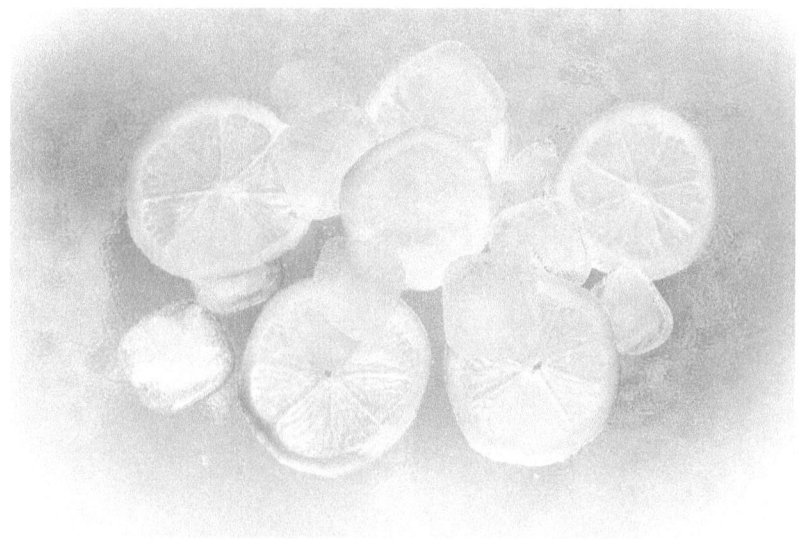

This chilly and zesty beverage is the perfect thing to sip when you're lounging poolside.

Ingredients

- Zest from 1 Lemon
- Juice from 2 Lemons
- 1 cup Sugar
- 4 cups Milk

Method

1. In a bowl, stir first 3 ingredients together. Stir in milk. Pour into a 9"x9" dish and freeze. Let chill 2 hours (stir once after 1 hour). Crush and pour into glasses.

26. Mango Sorbet

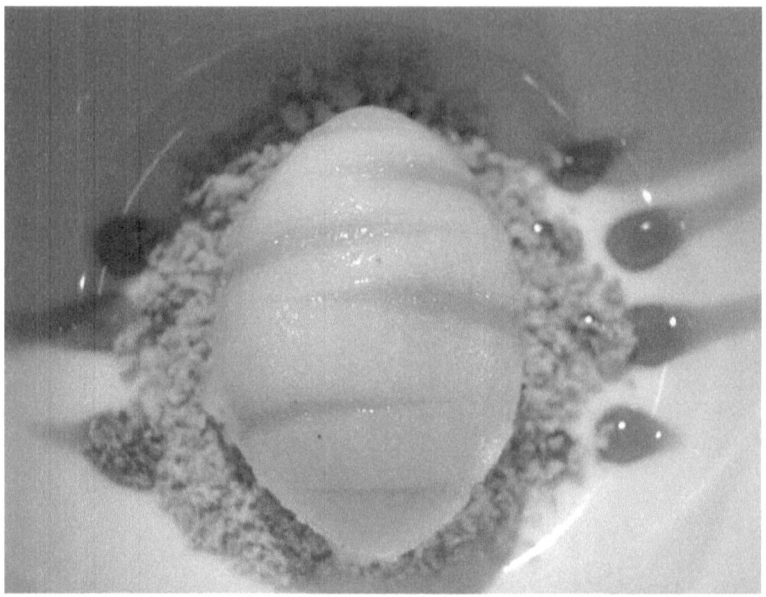

Make your own tropical sorbet with this simple recipe.

Ingredients

- 4 Mangoes (cubed)
- 1 cup Water
- 1 cup Sugar
- 3 Tbsps. Fresh Lime Juice

Method

1. In a small pot over medium-high heat, stir water and sugar until dissolved. Remove from heat. Puree mango in a food processor.

2. Add sugar mixture and lime juice. Pulse until combined. Place mixture into an ice cream maker and prepare according to directions.

27. Ice Cream Snow

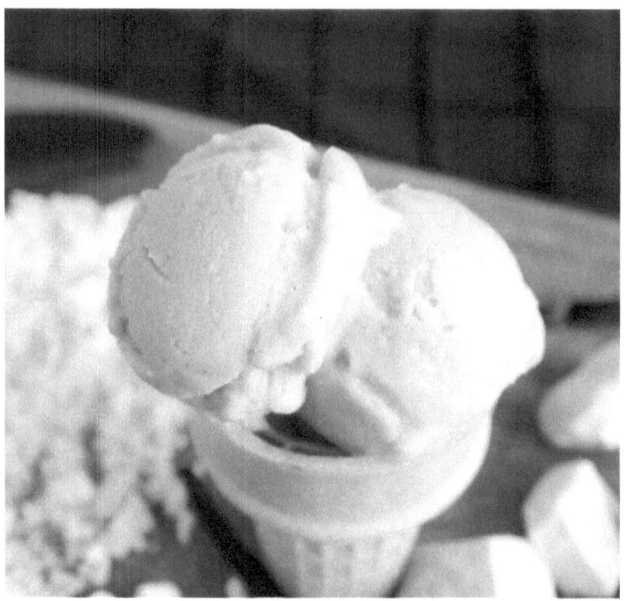

Stock up on fresh snow throughout the winter to make this delectable dessert come summer.

Ingredients

- 1-gallon Fresh Snow
- 1 cup Sugar
- 2 cups Milk
- 1 Tbsp. Vanilla Extract

Method

1. Stir ingredients together in a large serving bowl until well combined. Serve immediately.

28. Lime Coconut Sorbet

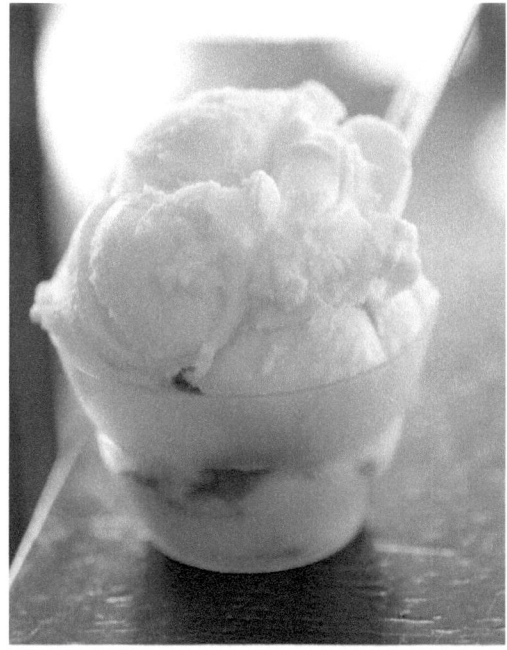

Lime gives this tropical sorbet a perfect hint of tanginess.

Ingredients

- 1 (15oz.) can Coconut Cream
- ¾ cup Water
- ½ cup Fresh Lime Juice

Method

1. Mix ingredients together in an ice cream maker. Prepare according to directions.

29. Creamy Avocado Pops

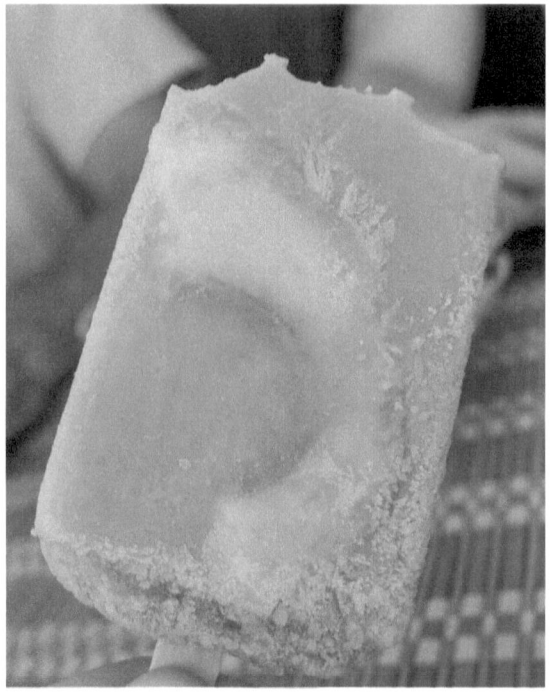

Avocado provides a rich creaminess and unique flavor to these summery treats.

Ingredients

- 3 Avocados (peeled, pitted)
- 1 cup Water
- ½ cup Sugar
- Juice from 1 Lime
- ¼ tsp Salt

Method

1. In a small pot, bring water and sugar to a boil. Stir constantly until dissolved. Remove from heat. Let cool.

2. In a blender, pulse everything together until smooth. Pour mixture into Popsicle molds. Freeze 2 hours. Insert sticks. Freeze overnight.

Final Words

I would like to thank you for downloading my book and I hope I have been able to help you and educate you about something new.

If you have enjoyed this book and would like to share your positive thoughts, could you please take 30 seconds of your time to go back and give me a review on my Amazon book page!

I greatly appreciate seeing these reviews because it helps me share my hard work!

Again, thank you and I wish you all the best with your cooking journey!

Disclaimer

This book and related site provides recipe and food advice in an informative and educational manner only, with information that is general in nature and that is not specific to you, the reader. The contents of this book and related site are intended to assist you and other readers in your personal efforts. Consult your physician or nutritionist regarding the applicability of any information provided in our information to you.

Nothing in this book should be construed as personal advice or diagnosis, and must not be used in this manner. The information provided about conditions is general in nature. This information does not cover all possible uses, actions, precautions, side-effects, or interactions of medicines, or medical procedures. The information in this site should not be considered as complete and does not cover all diseases, ailments, physical conditions, or their treatment.

No Warranties: The authors and publishers don't guarantee or warrant the quality, accuracy, completeness, timeliness, appropriateness or suitability of the information in this book, or of any product or services referenced by this site.

The information in this site is provided on an "as is" basis and the authors and publishers make no representations or warranties of any kind with respect to this information. This site may contain inaccuracies, typographical errors, or other errors.

Liability Disclaimer: The publishers, authors, and other parties involved in the creation, production, provision of information, or delivery of this site specifically disclaim any responsibility, and shall not be held liable for any damages, claims, injuries, losses, liabilities, costs, or obligations including any direct, indirect, special, incidental, or consequences damages (collectively known as "Damages") whatsoever and howsoever caused, arising out of, or in connection with the use or misuse of the site and the information contained within it, whether such Damages arise in contract, tort, negligence, equity, statute law, or by way of other legal theory.

www.ingramcontent.com/pod-product-compliance
Lightning Source LLC
Chambersburg PA
CBHW021132080526
44587CB00012B/1259